Six steps to a healthy, rich and fulfilling life

An immune system guide.

By

CINDY ZAHN

INTRODUCTION

The immune system is a very complex system of the human body. It acts as the body's defense against any infectious disease. If the body's immune system is at peak performance, it will have the ability to fight off any disease. If not, then your body will become more susceptible to any foreign invasion.

It is extremely important, I feel, to be able to lead a rich, healthy and fulfilling life. In order to do this your body must be running at peak performance. For your body to be at peak performance you need to have a healthy immune system.

Benjamin Franklin once said: "While we may not be able to control all that happens to use, we can control what happens inside us…" What he is suggesting is that while it is impossible at times to control the many things that happen, we do have some control over what happens inside our bodies. Our bodies are a reflection of our inner well-being. If we exercise and eat well, our bodies are going to perform well.

If we eat food that is not good for our bodies and forget to care for our bodies, fail to wash our hands or engage in other actions that promote disease, often we become sick.

This is your choice. Choose to treat your body right and it will reward. Choose to do what is not good for the body and pay the consequences.

The purpose of this book is to show you what the right choices are. You have the power in your hands for a rich, healthy fulfilling life. What will you do?

Table of Contents

Disclaimer

The information contained in this guide is for information purposes only. The author provides no warranty about the content or accuracy of content enclosed. Information contained herein is subjective. Keep this in mind when reviewing this guide.

The information in this guide is not provided as medical advice. You should always consult with your physician if you have a health condition that requires treatment. The author of this guide is not a medical doctor, psychologists or psychotherapists of any kind, and is not qualified to provide medical, psychological or therapeutic advice. You agree to hold all parties associated with creation and sales of this guide free from liability associated with any physical, mental, emotional, psychological or other harm arising from use of this guide.

CHAPTER 1. YOUR BODY UNDER ATTACK

No matter what time of year it is, your body is always subject to attack. It could be from the common cold, the flu, food poisoning or some other virus you contracted at work, school, or any other place you may frequent. Disease is everywhere. That doesn't mean you are defenseless to control diseases. There are many steps you can take to strengthen your immune system. What are these steps?

We'll talk more about them later. First, you have to know how disease works and when you are most likely to get sick. Once you understand this, everything else should fall into place. So, when are you most vulnerable to illness?

During winter people are more likely to become symptomatic mainly because they are inside. Without proper ventilation, anybody that stays inside for any length of time is subject to attack. Some people are also more sedentary in the winter than at other times during the year when the weather is warm and pleasing. If you find you are a couch potato during the cold winter months, you are probably more at risk for getting sick. Except if you follow proper hygiene habits and air out your home daily. Even if you do this, there is no guarantee that you will not get sick. If, however, your body is in good shape, you may be able to reduce the severity of your illness.

Anyone can become sick any time of the year, even during the warm summer months. While this may sound scary, there is some good news. Our body's immune system is always ready to fight foreign invaders. Unless your immune system is compromised (as is many times the case with persons who have autoimmune diseases) the chances are low that you will have to fight that virus you contracted at your office party for months on end.Most people, even those that do not use medicines, will get over the common cold and related viruses within a week to ten days.

If you do have a disease that compromises your immune system, you are more at risk for disease. But this does not mean you have to surrender to a disease. You can still fight back, and you should. The means you use to achieve good health however may be more rigorous than those offered in this guide alone. Be sure to talk to your healthcare provider if you suffer from a disease that makes it difficult for your immune system to fight the common cold and other foreign invaders.

There are many other organisms besides viruses that can attack your body, including bacteria. Fortunately, bacterial infections are normally curable with antibiotics. While medicine only decreases symptoms in most viral attacks, it will usually eliminate bacteria or the cause of occurrences in people with these types of conditions.

The problem with antibiotics

Antibiotics are at times considered a "panacea". This means that people think they are a form of medicine capable of killing all kinds of diseases. This is not true. While there are many antibiotics existing to treat disease, they are effective for killing diseases caused by bacteria, not those caused by a virus.

There is no antibiotic that helps cure a viral infection. If you take an antibiotic when you have a viral cold, you may build up antibodies. If your body later develops an illness due to a bacterial infection, the antibiotic your doctor may give to you might not work.

Bacteria are organisms that grow, change and mature. They are especially good at adapting. That means they can adapt to their surroundings, becoming more powerful. When this happens, many antibiotics that used to be able to cure an infection are no longer able to do so. At present there are not many antibiotics available to treat some of the more hazardous diseases. It seems like every year we are hearing about some "superbug" that is resistant to any current therapy. The main reason behind this is the constant use of antibiotics being prescribed. When you are constantly taking antibiotics, your body will eventual build up a resistance. This is mostly due to misuse of antibiotics. Many physicians feel pressured to prescribe them to patients that demand an antibiotic to feel better. The patient does not understand that sometimes the antibiotic may have a placebo effect, meaning that they start to feel better even though their recovery has nothing to do with the antibiotic. On the other hand, the person may feel better because by the time they take the antibiotic their body may already be effectively fighting the virus that first attacked their body.

Antibiotics are not something to fool around with. If you can find another suitable option, then use it. But check with your physician before doing so.

Now that you know how imperative it is to prevent illness and prepare your body to fight illness, let's see how you would go about doing just that.

Can you boost your immune system?

Yes, it is conceivable that you can strengthen your body so you are less likely to develop a cold. Or at the very least if you do get a cold your body will return to health faster than normal. This guide is a tool anybody can utilize to help fight back against the common cold, flu, bacterial diseases, food borne illness, poisoning and more. Please note before we continue, if you are sick you should always check in with your physician or other medical healthcare provider.

Your physician is the person in charge of your health. I have done my best to provide you with helpful and pertinent information in this guide; however, the author and publisher of this guide are not doctors. Remember that. If you are taking any medicine or being treated for a particular illness or chronic disease, speak to your doctor about any of the information given before you start using them.

Understood? Great! This book is a collection of years' worth of study into the human body and the link between mind, body and spirit. This is not about religion. What is meant is simple: by recognizing the reasons for illness rather than just treating the symptoms, you strengthen your mind, your physical body and your spirit, otherwise known as your gut or your subconscious.

All human body systems work in synchronization with each other, typically to help shield you from disease. While we can't infuse aromatherapy oils or vitamin C into the air filters at the job, we can provide you with solid information about tools people have used effectively to boost their immune systems. Remember that every person is unique. What works for one person may not work as effectively for another. You must find out what methods or tools work best for you and your body.

Always seek medical advice before attempting to treat or cure an illness

Remember, your physician is the one person that is most trained to diagnose an illness. Your physician can tell you if he or she suspects that you might have a viral or bacterial infection.

Now let's review the numerous tools available. These are tools anyone can use to help boost their immune system. The practices and tools in this guide do not come with a guarantee. They may not work for everyone. But, many people find these tools and methods are valuable and helpful for stopping disease or limiting the duration of a disease that already exists (like the common cold).

Are you ready to learn more?

You may find portions of this book more useful to you than others, so be sure to highlight them. You can at the very least make your own "to do" list if you discover something about immune boosting strategies you think will help you while you endeavor to defeat your illness.

CHAPTER 2. UNDERSTANDING YOUR IMMUNE SYSTEM

Before you learn how you can protect your immune system from foreign attackers, you must first know how your immune system works. When you understand this, you can use several tools, including visualization and meditation practices, to develop your body's health and capacity to defend against disease, no matter its origin.

The immune system is central to our livelihood. When we care for it right, it will do exactly as we want it to. Even if we get sick, when we are healthy most of the time, our body will react by fighting diseases and bacteria much harder. Now, let's take a look at our immune system and find out how it works.

Your internal bio-powered immune fighting machine

If we took impeccable care of our bodies, we would realize that our bodies are bio-powered immune fighting machines. It would be stronger than any antioxidant or antibiotic available. We are made to instinctively gather food, care for our loved ones and offspring, and fight against any attackers, whether visible or invisible to the human eye.

Our bodies were made to combat infection and disease.

How do our bodies do this? Let's discover how our body works to find any bacterial or viral agent that may enter.

Bacterial and viral agents can get into the body in many different ways. Just because you wash your hands a few times a day does not mean that you are safe.

Here are some examples that shows in a few simple steps what happens when disease enters your body.

1) Bacteria or viral organisms enter your body through touch, sneezes, physical contact or through other devices. When someone coughs, their phlegm may spread 500 feet. If they do not cover their mouth when they cough,

whatever illness they have will bathe the people around them. That is why it is so important to cover your mouth if you have to cough or sneeze.

2) Your body's immune system gets an indicator from your brain that calls out "time to make white blood cells!" White blood cells are the types of cells in your body that respond to infection. Their mission is to aid in creating cells that will fight disease whether they are viral or bacterial in nature.

3) Your body will also start to produce antibodies, which are specific kinds of white blood cells that fight off infection. Antibodies, including IgE, help to fight allergies and other conditions. IgA is a type of antibody that normally aids in the fight against infection.

4) If your immune system is running at peak performance, your body will direct adequate antibodies and white blood cells to fight any outbreak, no matter the severity. This doesn't mean you won't get sick. It means that your

body will do whatever it takes to keep you healthy. If you get sick, the odds are high that you will get well faster if your immune system is working wonders.

5) It may take a few days, but most people get better from minor infections or viruses rather quickly. It could take 7 to 10 days for the average cold or bacterial infection to resolve. Immuno-compromised patients may find it takes their body much longer to get rid of something as simple as the common cold.

Unfortunately, many people do not have a fine-tuned immune system. If you did, you probably wouldn't need to read this guide, would you? This guide will aid you in "fine tuning" your immune system so you have the greatest odds of decreasing the duration of an illness or stopping an illness all at the same time. Now that you know a little bit more about your immune system, it's time to learn about the many elements that may affect your immune system. These are things that may make your immune system operate less optimally than you would like.

CHAPTER 3. FACTORS THAT INFLUENCE YOUR IMMUNE SYSTEM

Your immune system may be compromised in many ways. Here are some reasons your body may not defend against an infection or disease the way you think it should.

If you engage in only one or two of these habits, they could affect your immune system adversely. Some people will fall ill even if their immune systems are attacked a little. Here are some examples.

- **You eat too much fast food or have too much saturated fat in your diet**. Fat can block your arteries, contribute to type II diabetes and increase the total body fat you carry around with you.
- **You hardly ever exercise, and when you do, you do it reluctantly, or you over do it, which can cause you to be sick instead of preventing illness**. Sometimes more is better; however, more is not better if you exercise to

the point where you over train your muscles and body. You need to give your body a break, especially between strength training sessions, so you are able to fight against disease.

- **You thrive on stress, which sends levels of cortisol (a stress hormone) skyrocketing, which can cause general malaise or illness**. Stress can be a killer. In fact, stress can lead to heart attack, high blood pressure, anger and hostility, depression and many other diseases. Your body will be better able to fight off disease if stress levels are low.

- **You don't get enough sleep, which can also alter the hormone levels in your body**. This makes you want to eat more and increases your vulnerability to common colds or infections. You may experience weight gain, which can also put you at risk for diseases like type II diabetes.

- **You sleep too much, which doesn't allow your body the physical activity it needs to get going and perform at its best**. It is necessary for you to sleep. But, if you are sleeping more than 10 hours a day, you may have a health problem. You should see your physician. Most people do well when they sleep 6-8 hours each day, preferably closer to the 7 to 8 hour range.

- **You either don't eat enough or you eat too much, so your body is not receiving the fuel it needs to fight disease**. The good news is that you don't have to deny yourself of all the rich foods that you like to be healthy; you just have to use a hands-on method, one that inspires self-control in all things. When you deny yourself food for too long, your body goes into starvation mode. This will actually slow down your metabolism, meaning you will gain weight even if you eat less than you have in the past

It sounds a bit technical, but when you look at your immune system as a complex machine, which it is, you are more likely to take care of and fine tune it. You would put oil in your car if it needed it, wouldn't you? The same is true here. You have to take care of your body just as you would any other appliance or other object that belongs to you (that you care about).

If you don't care for your body and do maintenance checks (annual physicals) you are more likely to get sicker than you might have been able to prevent. Your physician may find something in your blood tests that you didn't know about had you not visited him or her to begin with. You can do without many things in life. You can do without extra cheese on your cheeseburger; you can try spending a little less money. One thing you need to invest in however is your health. When your health is at its peak, you feel great. When you feel great, you can do almost anything your heart desires.

Now it's time for you to learn the steps needed to ensure your wellness. When you follow the steps given in the next chapter, you will be well on your way to a healthy, rich and fulfilling life. Are you ready? Then keep reading to discover what you need to do to take on the world with health and stamina.

CHAPTER 4. STEP BY STEP HEALTH ROUTINE

Your immune system is your best friend when you want to aid in protecting your body against colds, influenza and other common illnesses that often strike young children, the elderly and people with compromised immune systems. Remember, if you are not eating properly and getting some exercise, you might as well think of yourself as compromised.

Don't worry about labeling yourself; that isn't important. It is more important you know the steps you have to take to lead a healthier and cleaner life. Here is how you do that.

STEP 1: WASH YOUR HANDS

The first step is the simplest step to follow.

The number one way that people get sick is by hand-to-hand contact. You may shake the hand of somebody that is ill and fail to remember to wash your hands before you eat your lunch.

You may hold your child's hand while taking her to the park to play on the equipment. This equipment may contain several hundred different kinds of viruses or bacteria. Then when you return home, you fail to remember to wash your hands.

These are bad habits, very bad habits. These are the kind of habits that will cause you to become ill. You and every one in your family should always wash their hands, particularly if someone in the house is sick. Here are some times where it is critical for you to wash your hands.

- **Any time you go outside and return home**. This is particularly true if you go to busy places.
- **Any time you take your child to the park**. If you want to have a picnic and there is nowhere handy to wash your hands, then make sure you pack some moist towelettes. You can buy these almost anywhere. They are great for use when on-the-go. Another thing you might want to keep handy is a small bottle of hand

sanitizer. You can buy pocket sized sanitizer and give one to each member of the family. You just squeeze a tiny bit in your palms and rub them clean, no water or rinsing needed. Some even come with built in lotion or aloe to promote softness for your hands during cold winter months.

- **When you go out to eat**. Any time you go out to eat you should wash your hands before you eat your food. This is a setting where you can simply use a moist towel or take a trip to the restroom to clean up before you eat.

- **When caring for a loved one that is ill**. At times while taking care of the people we love, we overlook how important it is to care for ourselves. However, illness can be spread by caring for somebody who is sick and then touching another person if you do not wash your hands.

- **When handling pets or pet material**. Pets are nice to have, but they often harbor many diseases. Make sure you wash your hands after touching the family dog.

- **Before planning and preparing meals**. You should always wash your hands before and after handling food products you plan to eat or to serve others. If you are sick, you may contaminate everybody in the home. Be especially cautious when cooking food that includes meat and vegetables. Raw meat may harbor many diseases including salmonella or E. coli. Be sure that you do not use the same cutting board for preparing vegetables and then use it for the meat. Each should have its own special cutting board.

STEP 2 – EAT IMMUNE BOOSTING FOODS

There are a lot of immune boosting foods that you can eat. These foods will not cure a cold instantaneously, but they may make your body able to fight harder against disease.

Most people know that fruits, whole grains and vegetables top the list of must eat items. Some people think that chicken soup makes you feel better when you are sick. Other people still live by the old adage "starve a cold and feed a fever."

So what should you eat? Here is a list of the foods that are most likely to result in better health. These foods have shown to be helpful in boosting one's total wellness, which in turn might help to boost the odds you will be able to fight infection or viruses if they attack.

- **Fish or Flax** – these foods deliver essential fatty acids, which are tiny substances that are great for decreasing inflammation in the body, which is a common cause of illness. While you can take a supplement containing Omega-3 fatty acids (a key essential fatty acid) you can also get essential fatty acids from your diet. Some good sources of fatty acids in food include fatty fishes like tuna, salmon and mackerel.

- **Yogurt** – yogurt contains ingredients called probiotics that help balance the flora in the digestive tract. When the flora in the body becomes out of control, diseases like yeast infections or UTI become common.

- **Mushrooms** – Eastern medical doctors often use Shitake mushrooms to boost the immune system. Most mushrooms contain vitamin B and other essential nutrients. You will benefit whether you eat the Shitake kind or any other kind, as long as you include them into an overall healthy diet.

- **Fresh fruits** – especially blueberries, strawberries and bananas. All of these contain powerful ingredients to boost the immune system and aid the body in fighting back against disease. Blueberries, raspberries and strawberries contain many antioxidants; these are substances that reduce free radical damage. Free radical damage is damage that occurs on the surface of an object. Free radical damage can occur from too much unprotected exposure to the sun or other environmental pollutants. Bananas contain plenty of potassium, which helps balance the electrolytes in your body.

- **Seaweed** – some believe seaweed (often used in Eastern dishes like sushi) contains ingredients that boosts the action of T cells in the body; these are disease fighting cells. Seaweed may also cause the body to make more antibodies, which are a type of white blood cell that helps fight disease and infection.
- **Herbs** – herbs are potent ingredients anybody can utilize to flavor dishes and fight disease. There are certain herbs like cumin, cayenne and cilantro that may help boost circulation and improve one's immunity. This is particularly true of cayenne, which heats the body. Some believe cayenne may help increase the metabolism also, which is why it is an ingredient in many natural health supplements promoting weight loss benefits.

- **Green Tea** – this tea, like many other teas, is a dynamo of antioxidants. Black tea also holds a lot of useful antioxidants, but research suggest that green tea is best. You can buy it decaf or caffeinated. Green tea is often used in weight loss products because many believe it stimulates the metabolic system. The antioxidants in the tea may help ward off infection or illness. Sipping tea with a bit of honey and lemon while sick can soothe an itchy, red or sore throat.

- **Water** – it may sound silly, but a lot of people mistake thirst for hunger and overeat. Water, pure, filtered and clean water is one of the best substances you can drink if you want to stay well or get better faster. Water hydrates the body. Most people do not drink enough water. Water is essential for every biological process that occurs in the body. Water helps the digestive system work properly

It helps your skin feel healthy and it helps your body recover from illness. If you don't like the taste of water, there are many products now promoting water with added flavors you can try. Just be sure to stay away from those that have a lot of calories or you might experience some weight gain. If you are dehydrated however, some people find an electrolyte enhanced drink like Gatorade or similar products help replenish the system. You can even drink some water with a pinch of sea salt and lemon to help balance the electrolytes in your body.

- **Garlic and Onion** – fresh garlic has many immune boosting properties, whether you take it as a supplement or as a whole food. If you get fresh garlic and fry it or add it to favorite foods including sauces, you will give your immune system a power boost. Garlic has antifungal, antibacterial and energy boosting qualities. When combined with onion in light broth, many people find it helps relieve sinus congestion or lessens the amount of time they suffer from a cold. When in doubt, always go for the garlic, and take a breath freshener with you while out and about.

- **Oats and Barley** – These are whole grains having lots of a healthy fiber that contains antioxidants and antimicrobial ingredients. Many people believe that oats and barley are more beneficial then Echinacea. Some studies propose that oats and barley may be helpful for people who have compromised immune systems, or those that are prone to the flu and related illnesses.

This list is far from complete, but it does give you an idea of the kinds of foods you can eat that are most likely to result in better health. You should think about eating whole foods rather than processed or packaged foods, as many processed foods (even if fortified with vitamins) contain too much fat and too many preservatives.

Whole foods include those that are in their complete state. They are natural, minimally processed and good for you. You can find grains, vegetables and lean proteins that are whole foods. Look for meat that does not contain antibiotics. A lot of processed meats from traditional stores are loaded with hormones to help the cows providing the meat and milk to grow.

These hormones do not vanish. If you give your child whole milk that has been pasteurized and comes from a cow that feeds on antibiotics or growth hormones, your child may be ingesting the same hormones. Some scientists consider this is one of the reasons why so many young adolescents are hitting puberty much earlier in life.

You can even have organic foods prepared and delivered right to your door. Many organizations deliver boxed goods containing a wide variety of organic products.

You can also order pre-cooked meals online. Here is an example of a site that does just that:

www.theorganicdish.com

It's just like any other prepared food service, like weight watchers, however with this program you get organic ingredients and meals delivered right to your door. You may also look in your local phone book, as many organizations like this are sprouting in small and large cities that have an inclination toward natural and organic foods and lifestyles.

STEP 3 – TAKE YOUR VITAMINS & SUPPLEMENTS

Eating well is vital to your health; so is taking the right vitamins and supplements. During various stages of our life we all need a little extra spark. You should always talk with your healthcare provider before you use any over-the-counter supplement.

This is particularly true if you take prescription medicines on a regular basis because some supplements or vitamins may adversely interact with each other. Some supplements may increase or reduce the side effects of prescription medicines, as can some foods. So be sure you talk to your doctor before you try any of these.

A trained healthcare provider can also guide you by telling you how much of a vitamin or supplement you need to take to attain improved health or to boost your immune system.

Here is a list of some of the more common supplements recommended to people for boosting the immune system.

- **Probiotics** – Sometimes referred to as "acidophilus", probiotics help balance the natural flora or good bacteria that exist in in the body. Often when someone takes antibiotics, the antibiotic kills off all bacteria in the body, both good and bad. Good bacteria are necessary for proper digestion and elimination. Some studies advise that the use of probiotics in children and in adults may lower digestive disease risk, improve immunity to common diseases and may even lower the number of infectious diseases that cause fever in people that take them regularly.

- **Omega-3 fatty acid** – is a supplement containing omega-3 like fish oil or flax seed oil and may improve your overall health and wellness. Essential fatty acids like this also help reduce inflammation in the body. Often physicians recommend patients with arthritis or similar diseases take an anti-inflammatory agent like essential fatty acids.

- **Vitamin C** – vitamin C is one of the least expensive and easiest ways to get your daily serving of immune boosting ingredients. There is much debate in the health community about how much vitamin C is enough vitamin C to defend the body. One way to determine this is to take one tablet a day, and increase your dose until you feel abdominal discomfort. However, this may not work for all people. It is best you speak with your healthcare professional about the proper dose of vitamin C for you based on your health and body weight.

- **Echinacea** – this herb has been promoted as a virtual panacea for all illnesses. If taken frequently during a cold it may help lessen the length or severity of a cold. You can buy it as an herb, in capsule or tincture preparations. Many healthcare providers recommend you do not take this year 'round, as it may lose its ability to fight disease if taken every day. If you are ill, you might consider taking it for a week and then taking a week off to see how well you do. Studies about Echinacea are controversial; some people swear by its effectiveness and others doubt it helps at all. Remember, all bodies are different. If you take it and it seems to help, then use it. If you find it doesn't then try something else.

- **Goldenseal** – this is a potent herb that you should use with care. Manufacturers note it has antibacterial and antiseptic properties. It can cause digestive upset, and should not be taken during pregnancy as it can stimulate contractions or early labor. Goldenseal is a species that is dying out. It is vital to take it when needed, and to take only as much as you need to feel better. A skilled herbalist can work with you to find out what the best dose is for your body type.

- **Zinc** – many people have zinc deficiencies which may cause fatigue and lethargy. Many cold formulas at stores now offer zinc as a primary ingredient. This is true of many tablets used to soothe a sore throat. It is sometimes difficult to get enough zinc from the food you eat, so if you are sick you may find it helps to take a little extra zinc. Often you can find a zinc lozenge.

If you want to know more about supplements and herbs that may help to bolster your immune system, you should think about locating a trained natural healthcare provider or consult with an herbalist before you buy anything.

You will discover that there are many other supplements on the market that claim they boost health and wellness. Some of these contain a mixture of ingredients or herbs and natural vitamins and minerals. Before you purchase a supplement after hours of searching the shelves of a health food store, talk with a trained herbalist or other health care practitioner. He or she can help you decide what, if any, supplement will help you best as you try to overcome your illness. Only someone that is qualified and comprehends basic anatomy and physiology, and the drug interactions likely to happen when somebody takes an herb with a medicine, can really assist you as you try to find the best immunity formula to suit your needs.

You can also ask what herbs you can use or foods you can use to help prevent disease (like shitake mushrooms and seaweed). Some foods and supplements (including garlic) are sometimes better taken as a preventive medicine than as a cure for any illness.

Speaking of garlic, you may also want to think about adding more garlic to your diet, whether in the form of a capsule or raw garlic. Garlic acts in much the same way that goldenseal does; many consider it natures natural antibiotic. Be careful not to eat too much at once though as it may upset your stomach. And many newer supplements containing garlic are now odorless and tasteless. So no worries about garlic breath.

Now that you have an idea of what types of supplements you can take to improve your immunity, let's look at the next two steps you can take to help your immune system punch out disease.

STEP 4 – EXERCISE

You knew it would arise at some point, the great sermon on exercise. First, don't think of this as a sermon. This book is a tool you can use to help improve your health and wellness. It is not something that you should dread. Everyone needs to exercise.

I will not be telling you how you will exercise or what type of exercising is best for you. You are better off talking to your physician about that question. I can however, let you in on a secret – a little exercise will boost your immune system. That's true whether you exercise one hour a day or 10 minutes 7 days a week.

Even if you are thin, you may need to get more exercise. Many people think that because they are thin that they do not need to exercise much to stay in shape. However, quite the opposite is true. There are many "thin" people walking around that are "fat" on the inside, and the inside is what counts. You can have a high body fat percentage and still "look" skinny. Why is this? Muscle weighs more than fat.

Someone that is 120 pounds and 14% lean looks very different from someone that is 120 pounds and has 30 % body fat. The person with 30 percent body fat may be just under five feet tall, but based on the body fat calculation they are obese.

If you want a true measure of how healthy you are, which predicts your odds of staying in great shape and fighting disease, you should ask your doctor to do a body fat measurement and BMI calculation.

Once you find out what these numbers are, you can start a practical exercise program, say 20 minutes of exercise three days each week. In time, you will discover that exercise is pleasing and you can work your way up the ladder, working out 30 minutes instead of 20 minutes. The progression continues.

BMI stands for body mass index. It is a tool many physicians and therapists use to measure how fit or unfit a person's body is. There are many free calculators you can use on the web to determine your body mass index, including ones from the Centers for Disease Control, American Heart Association, and National Institutes of Health.

Here are a couple of links you can follow to learn more:

CDC Adult & Child BMI Calculators
www.cdc.gov/nccdphp/dnpa/bmi - this is a great site with a lot of free information on computing BMI and fat mass for children and adults. You can also find out more about the many different diseases there are that are

susceptible to weight changes. You may also learn more about infectious diseases and how to prevent them.

Adult BMI Calculator UK

www.health.nsw.gov.au/obesity/adult/bmi.html

As with any calculator this allows you to calculate your BMI in kilograms or in pounds if you convert the figures. This site also offers information on childhood obesity and tips for overcoming obesity and overweight.

Youth BMI Calculator UK

www.health.nsw.gov.au/obesity/youth/bmi.html

This is a good tool for parents interested in finding out how healthy their child is. You can use the tool on this page to calculate the BMI for children and young adults to age 18. It is important to note calculations for young children are different from those adults use.

The National Institute of Health also offers a written clarification of how to calculate your body mass index manually. While many people prefer the old' calculator, may physicians and healthcare providers will calculate BMI manually or use a special "map" of the human body that outlines or separates healthy weights from unhealthy weights. If you want to find out what your BMI is manually just follow the formula below.

1. First, weigh yourself, write that number down.
2. Next, multiply your weight in pounds by the number 703.
3. Now, divide the answer you get by your height (calculated in inches).
4. Finally, divide the answer from step 3 by your height again (in inches).

This is a long but not hard method. If you want quick information you may find the BMI online calculators much faster.

You can measure your body fat with calipers, which most physicians and physical trainers have. There are other ways of calculating body fat, but most are long and burdensome. Most physicians or physical therapists offer body fat testing if asked. If they do not, find someone that does or ask your doctor for a referral. You can buy your own caliper online. If you do, remember you may have trouble differentiating fat from muscle mass or skin.

This means you are more likely to get an imprecise reading if you measure your body fat alone, unless you are already a health professional well-versed in body fat calculations. The BMI with the body fat analysis is the best predictor of health for most people. The BMI is often not the best choice for athletes because they may weigh a lot and still look skinny, resulting from the higher than average muscle mass in their bodies.

What exercises boost the immune system?

So far we have discussed everything EXCEPT the exercises you can take part in to boost your immune system. There are many exercises that anybody can take part in and have a good time.

The kind of exercise you choose will be subject to many things including your current health, your medical history and your physical activity history. If you have never exercised a day in your life, your best bet may be walking. While this seems controversial it is not. The more people walk, the more likely they are to be healthy.

When you walk for exercise you should walk as fast as you can, almost to the point where you are jogging, so you get your heart rate up, provided this is safe for you. You can pump your arms to increase the effects your walking has on your health.

You should ask your physician or other healthcare provider for some advice when power walking so you

know how long to walk and whether you can enjoy other exercises besides walking. Here is a list of exercises people commonly enjoy. These will help keep you in shape which naturally will help improve your ability to fight off infection.

1. **Swimming** – light swimming is great because it is easy on the joints and works every muscle group. If you are not able to swim you can still get in the pool and enjoy an aqua aerobics or related class to help you get in the swing of things.

2. **Stair Climbing** – provided you have strong knees you can climb outdoors where the air is fresh. If you have a school with a football stadium near you climb up and down the stairs on a nice day.

3. **Walking or Jogging** – many people find they start walking and eventually end jogging. Jogging on a grassy surface or other soft terrain (sand or soil) is easier on the knees than walking on pavement.

4. **Biking** – you can bike indoors or out. Try a reclined bike which allows you to sit in a way that doesn't harm your body. This type of cycle allows you to sit at an angle instead of straight up and down, so it is much easier to stay on the bike for long sessions.

5. **Strength Training** – this is an important part of any exercise program especially if you want to lose fat and improve your muscle mass. You can start out using machines and graduate to free weights. Make sure you have someone show you how to do an exercise correctly before you try doing something yourself. You may end up sorry if you don't. Strength training can be fun and exciting, but not if you tear a muscle.

6. **Yoga** – yoga is a great form of exercise that can improve your immunity and help improve your body's flexibility. Many of the poses are cleansing and gentle, ideal for someone that would like a moving meditation.

7. **Pilates** – like yoga, is a great exercise that can boost the body's immune system and lengthen muscles. You can work to correct muscle imbalances and realize greater strength.

8. **Tai Chi** – this is a meditative practice much like yoga but is much gentler, allowing the person participating to enjoy a standing meditation

while also moving in gentle postures and flow. Tai Chi purportedly can help restore the natural alignment of energies in the body.

9. **Meditation** – many people do not think of meditation as exercise. That's because they are looking at meditation wrong. Meditation is exercise; it is exercise for the body, mind and soul. When we allow ourselves to meditate, we feed our minds and provide our body with a chance to rest, relax and refresh. It also lowers stress, which is necessary if you want to improve your immunity to common ailments.

10. **Visualization** – exercises for the mind include visualization exercises. You can imagine your body fighting back against disease. Just close your eyes, create an image of your perfect, healthy body, and hold that vision close to your mind and heart. The mind is very powerful. When we believe that in using our minds we are well and free of disease, most times our bodies respond accordingly.

Your body, mind and spirit need daily exercise to survive. If you focus on disease, then you are more prone to disease. What you should be doing is concentrating on health and conquering disease. Cancer patients are often taught visualization skills that help them overcome their disease. Cancer is a disease where abnormal cells grow out of control.

Gentle motions done through Tai Chi, Yoga or a practice called Qigong (another type of Eastern exercise involving low-impact movement of energy) are sometimes more helpful for boosting immunity than vigorous exercise, which may actually increase the stress hormones circulating in your system. Gentle motion exercises as these are helpful for providing your body with more energy, which means you have more ability to fight off infection and feel your best. You can enjoy these exercises as much or as little as you want.

You can visualize disease or a chronic illness any way you want. The goal is to focus on getting rid of the cells responsible for your disease or the virus and bacteria accountable for your fatigue. You can also perform visualizations where you imagine what your body would look like in a healthy state. You can imagine your perfect body, and then imagine you accomplishing any task you want with your perfect body. Many people with strong immune systems imagine their body is healthy whether it is or not.

Your subconscious can "trick" your brain into thinking you are healthy even if you are not healthy. It sounds strange, but it can happen. Physicians are using visualization techniques in hospitals to help patients recover faster. There are even studies suggesting visualization helps improve medical health and outcomes among patients with chronic illnesses.

It is really a matter of mind over matter – in a literal way.

Those opposing such techniques suggest visualization offers nothing more than what a placebo would. The placebo effect is the feeling of something positive changing without anything actually changing. This can happen for many reasons. If people are given a medication and told it will cure their disease, they are more likely to realize positive health outcomes whether or not they receive medicine or a sugar pill (at least in some cases).

The placebo effect does not happen for everyone, but it might work for you, even if you do not believe in visualizations to boost your immunity. What is the worst thing that can happen? You may end up right where you started, or you may find you feel a thousand times better.

Step 5 – Reduce Stress

If you decrease the amount of stress you carry with you, you are more likely to feel better. Stress is a prominent cause of illness in the United States and many others. It is important that you understand how much stress can impact your life.

When you feel stressed, usually you have difficulty sleeping. If you cannot sleep, then you cannot function well throughout your day and are more likely to become sick because your immune system is weak. With proper sleep and little stress, your body is much more likely to respond positively and overcome any illness that may come its way.

How much stress do you carry around in your life?

Before we go further, let's do a stress inventory. We are going to find out what you stress triggers are or how much stress you carry around with you daily. This can help to better your quality of life and health. Here are some common stress triggers. How many can you identify with?

1. Feeling tired or lethargic during the day even after a good night's sleep.

2. Worrying constantly about work assignments, school assignments or other activities that have a deadline.

3. Always arriving late to an event or meeting because you are scrambling to catch up on work that might have been done already had you not procrastinated.

4. You drink almost every night in excess to relax after a hard day's work.

5. Crying a lot for no reason, or feeling the "blues" constantly.

6. Falling behind your peers.

7. Driving recklessly or endangering yourself while driving or engaging in other ordinary activities.

8. Feeling irritable or angrier than usual.

9. Having trouble falling or staying asleep at night.

10. Feeling like simple task are overly cumbersome.

How many of these circumstances can you relate to? Stress is something you want to remove from your life as best you can. While you can't possibly rid the world of everything stressful, you can eliminate some of your stress, and some stress relief is better than no stress relief

Here are some tips you can implement to help release or reduce some of the stress in your life. The less stress you have the better your chance of fighting a cold. Remember, none of these practices guarantees you will not get sick; if you do get sick however, if you follow the advice offered in this guide you are more likely to recover much faster than others.

- **Plan ahead**. If you have to go to work the next day, then pick out what you want to wear the night before, and make sure it is ironed and pressed so you are ready to go. That way you can sleep in or hit the snooze button at least once without running late.

- **Exercise daily.** You don't have to be a marathon runner to reap the benefits of exercise. All you really have to do is get outside for 15 minutes once or twice a day. Exercise helps boost your body's immune system. When you exercise, you also feel better on the inside.

- **Organize and Prioritize**. If you have too much to do, you will find your tasks weigh you down. This can lead to stress, and stress contributes to illness. The most common argument people offer for not organizing is "I don't' have time". The reality is you do have time, especially if you want to get well. The less attention you pay to your body the more likely you are to stay sick. As long as you stay sick, you are going to suffer. If you take just 30 minutes out of each day to organize and prioritize, you will find your day flows much smoother. If you need help organizing, you can always ask a friend or family member to help out.

Naturally there are many other ways you can reduce stress. You can take a walk twice daily outside to get out of the house or your office building. You can take a 15-minute power nap. A power nap isn't really a nap. It is a small period of time you can use to recline, relax and kick back. The goal is not to think about the work ahead of you. Rather, you should spend the time focusing on creating more energy in your life. Imagine what your life would be like if you finished all of your tasks ahead of schedule. Once you do this, you are better able to manage the stress you do have on your plate without releasing too much in the way of cortisol or stress hormones.

Some people prefer traditional stress busters like a massage, pedicure or drive along the countryside. Any of these are a good idea. When you prepare for bed, try not to drink up to four hours before your head hits the pillow. While you may "think" the alcohol relaxes you, in the longer term it actually deprives you of much needed sleep. Alcohol only causes you to feel sleepy for a short time. Then it acts more like a stimulant, depriving you of deep sleep. You also develop a headache or become dehydrated, which can lead to even more stress.

You might consider setting up a bedtime ritual that involves meditation, a good read and silky sheets to relax in. Do whatever it is that appeals most to you to get the quality sleep you need.

STEP 6 – GET MORE SLEEP

Sleep is the best gift you can give your body. Many people are more prone to colds, flu, viruses, bacterial infections and chronic fatigue when they don't get enough sleep. There are many ways lack of sleep can affect your immune system. Let's look at some of them and come up with some common interventions that may help you to get a better nights' sleep.

Trouble sleeping

Many people have trouble falling or staying asleep. Often people have trouble falling asleep because:

> **They have too much on their mind**. To avoid going to sleep with a full head, begin a journal you can review at night to help you let go of your worries before bed. You can't solve anything while sleeping, so put your worries to rest before you put yourself to bed.
> **They drink before bed.** Drinking before bed is a big mistake. Make sure you take your last (alcoholic) drink at least four hours before going to bed. Avoid caffeinated beverages up to six hours before you go to sleep. This will make an obvious change in the way you sleep.

They exercise too close to bedtime. The best time to exercise is first thing in the morning. Exercise in the morning gives your metabolism a boost for the day, and then allows you to sleep better at night. If you exercise too close to bedtime, you will feel too charged to sleep.

They watch television in bed. The worst place to work or watch television is in bed. While it may "seem" comfy, it can create disaster on your sleep. Some studies propose that the light from a television or the light emitted by a computer is enough to give a person chronic insomnia. This light tricks your brain into thinking it is time to wake up, so you have a harder time sleeping.

They eat too much protein before bed. Protein is good for building muscle and boosting energy. If you want to sleep and stay asleep however, you might want to try a low protein high carbohydrate snack sometime within the hour or two before going to bed.

Make sure you do not eat too much before bed as this too can affect your sleep. A small snack however, may help keep your blood sugar levels aligned so you sleep better and longer. Most people discover that if they eat enough before bed that they do not wake nearly as often during the night.

They suffer jet lag. If you are a frequent flyer jet lag may be the cause of your insomnia. To help with this, ask your doctor about taking a melatonin supplement. This sometimes helps restore normal sleep patterns. But that can vary from person to person. I find that melatonin has the exact opposite effect on me. I took it one time and I could not get to sleep at all. You can also try altering your sleep schedule while on business or vacation so you do not mess up your normal sleep cycle rhythms. This may mean going to bed one or two hours earlier or later than normal, but most people would agree the change is worth it. Jet lag among frequent flyers is a concern and almost disabling problem if not handled correctly.

If you think that you don't have time to sleep, then you had better think again. Sleep is not an option. You must sleep. If you use the excuse that you have no time to sleep, then you need to work on your schedule and make more time for sleep. There's no such thing as "catching up" on sleep, so don't think that you can get in extra sleep during the weekends and work while sleep deprived during the week. It just doesn't work that way. You have to commit to a regular sleep routine to get acceptable results. If you do not have a sleep routine, then you had better consider creating one. Being sleep deprived will definitely take a toll on your immune system.

Your goal is to get seven to eight hours of sleep preferably, although some people can get by with only six to seven hours and others on eight to nine hours. Get to know your body, so you can decide how much sleep gets you where you need to be. You want to be feeling healthy and energetic throughout the day.

Sleep is a powerful tool. When we get enough sleep our bodies are better prepared to take on stress and disease. You will find you can overcome colds and infections much easier when you are fully rested. Make sure you sleep as much as you can especially when you are sick. You may find you need one or two extra hours of sleep when sick each day until better.

If this is true, get some sleep. Call in to work and tell them you are sick, whether you have sick time or not. Most managers and companies would prefer to have you working at peak capacity rather than spreading

disease throughout the company. Chances are high if you work while ill you will only escalate the severity of your disease. You could then face a potentially severe infection, especially if you expose your debilitated immune system to bacteria and pollutants on the job. Have you ever watched someone as they try to work while sick? Every sniffle and cough puts another person at risk for falling ill. Point that out to your manager if they give you trouble about staying home because of an illness.

Chapter 5. Conclusion

Congratulations! You are now on your way to healthy living. Caring for your body is one of the best steps you can take to wellness and an exceptional quality of life. Make sure you take care of your body as you would care for a child. You only get one chance to live in the skin you are currently in. There is no reason you need to damage your body to enjoy life.

Winter and spring are often the times when people become ill, usually resulting from viral infections or allergies. Make sure you get an annual or bi-annual check-up around these times so you can work with your physician to prevent disease and illness, rather than just treat it. If you live a healthy lifestyle on a regular basis, the chances are high you will feel and look your best, day in and day out.

In step 4 – exercise, I have books out on some of these exercise topics that you might want to check out. And those that I haven't gotten to yet, will be forthcoming in the future. Please check out my "Other books by Cindy Zahn" section of this book.

So now that you have completed this book, what are you going to do? Are you going to continue on as before, or are you going to take what you have learned to heart? You have the power in your hands for a rich, healthy and fulfilling life. What will you do?

ABOUT THE AUTHOR

Hello, my name is Cindy Zahn. I graduated from the Institute for Integrative Nutrition as a certified health coach. I also have three certificates from the Doctor Sears Wellness Institute in Prime Time Health (Adults & Seniors), Lean Expectations (Pregnant Woman and new Moms) and Lean Start (Young Families).

My passion is helping people to be able to live a rich, healthy and fulfilling life through eating the right foods, exercise and, when necessary, supplementation.

You can follow me on my Facebook author page: https://www.facebook.com/cszbestsellingauthor/ or through my whole foods lifestyle page: https://www.facebook.com/Your-whole-food-lifestyle-starts-here-109020742787635/.

For those of you who have purchased this book, I am giving you the opportunity to get a free 30-minute coaching session. Just send me an email at cindyzahn@gmail.com. I will try to respond with 24 hours. In the subject line please type "request for free consultation" so that I know you want to schedule a coaching session.

OTHER BOOKS BY CINDY ZAHN

Don't just sit there! Strength training for women.

Don't just sit there! Fitness walking for all ages.

Don't just sit there! How to get fit in 15 minutes a day.

Don't just sit there! The best way to learn yoga from home in 15 minutes a day for 21 days.

Don't just sit there! Start yoga for seniors now.

Hunger hormones: Top 10 questions answered.

The healing power of whole food.

The souper diet.

Healing foods of the Bible.

The amazing apple: A wholefood wonder

www.ingramcontent.com/pod-product-compliance
Lightning Source LLC
Chambersburg PA
CBHW062118280526
45788CB00003B/1505